An Angel

With

Blue Hair

By

Mary Michele McCarville

Exodus 23:20

Behold, I send an Angel before thee, to keep thee in the way, and to bring thee

into the place which I have prepared.

For

Jessica & Darren

I am a native of Arizona, living in Cave Creek in the beauty of the desert. I was born on October 2; the feast of the guardian angels and love angel stories. When my son Tommy was born, his name was to be Michael, after the most powerful angel. However, my husband filled out the birth certificate wrong and as fate has it, his name is Thomas Michael. Tommy met singles in his area on an app called *Tinder* and I noticed he was spending more time than usual with a girl he called "Al". I asked him what she was like and he said "edgy". I realized what he meant by that when I first met her, she had blue hair.

Al is beautiful, reminding me of a young Norma Jean, I often call her Marilyn. Tommy and Al bonded with love of music, traveling to concerts. One concert they attended was *Life is Beautiful* in the fall of 2015. During a break, they passed by a *Get on the List* table, a campaign to sign up for bone marrow transplant donor matches. They donated cheek swabs to join the registry and proudly put red and white *Bone Marrow Donor* cards in their wallets.

Several months later Al received a phone call. She was a probable match for a 4-month-old baby with blood cancer. The caller explained in detail the process of donating bone marrow, asking Al if she would consider the procedure. She said yes. She said yes right away.

She did not ask them if she could call them back after she thought about it. She did not consider the issues anyone would think about, the physical, mental and off from work cost if you did not feel well after the procedure. She immediately said yes and prepared herself to save a life, the life of a baby. She had a blood test locally to confirm she was a match, she was. She now was to have a preliminary exam to see if she could tolerate the surgery, and make sure she had no infectious diseases. She flew at no cost to her by air to spend a night in a hotel next to a hospital. My son Tommy was worried and insisted on going with her. The next morning they walked to the hospital. All day they went up and down the elevator to the different floors for various tests, such as blood work, X-Rays and EKG. Al was in perfect health; the surgery was scheduled.

When Tommy told me what Al was going to do, I was amazed. She is only 19 years old! Where did this young girl obtain such compassion? How could she have learned to love humanity, giving herself to others to this degree? I knew she loved animals. I had seen her rescue a stray dog she named "Kit" spending hours trying to catch her, taking her home for a bath, providing all the love and care a dog would ever need.

Al asked me at Christmas time if I would like to contribute to her mother's project to raise clothes and food for needy families. Her mother Jessica raised truckloads of donations delivering them herself to many needy families. I was starting to learn how Al learned how to give. Al spent her early years with her father Darren who stayed home with her, providing 24/7 care until she was old enough to attend grade school. Al says he taught her independence and courage.

Eleven years ago her mother starting working at a children's hospital where many terminally ill children go for medical care. Al grew up helping her mother with different events at the hospital, watching children walking down the hall pushing their IV poles, with colorful hats covering their baldheads.

Al and Tommy were flown at no cost to another state with a town car meeting them at the airport. The felt awkwardly important when a young handsome driver in a black suit held up a sign with Al's name. He drove them to a nice hotel to stay free with meals included for three nights. The hotel is within walking distance to the hospital. I flew in and met Al's mother Jessica who had driven from Phoenix. She wanted to make sure a vehicle was available for any issues that would arise. We went to dinner, Al picked Italian.

We had fun walking to a local Italian restaurant. During dinner, Al mentioned Nurse Laura told her the parents of the baby with blood cancer had the option of contacting Al by phone before the surgery. Al waited with great anticipation for the phone call, thinking about what they were going to say to each other. She waited and waited. The call never came. I could see the disappointment in her face. I thought to myself things would be easier for Al if they had called.

Al had to stop eating at midnight, we joked as she devoured pasta, chocolate cake and gelato. We arrived back at the hotel and Al announced she had one hour to keep eating and wanted chips. We ran laughing to the gift shop in the hotel before it closed. As Jessica paid for junk food, Al rested her face against her mother's chest and they hugged, crushing the chips against each other.

Through her smile, I could see the worry on Jessica's face. The hospital was next door, Al was to meet Nurse Laura there at six. Al was concerned we would be late. She announced she was going to set her alarm for 4:30 am to make sure we all made it on time. We reassured her that was much too early and agreed to meet in the lobby at 5:20 AM. I woke at 4:30 am for no reason. Al had won, I was up. I walked to the deserted lobby looking for coffee. None was to be found. It was dark outside and there was an odd steely feel in the air. I plopped down in a chair wondering why I felt like I was back in college about to take a final exam.

Jessica came toward me, shaking her beautiful hair full of tendrils in dismay, she had not slept. I told her not to bother looking for coffee. Tommy's tall handsome frame came into view with little Al attached to him like a glove, gripping his hand, hard. She announced she had not slept at all; Tommy had fallen asleep and snored in her ear. Tommy told us later Al was extremely anxious during the night and he had to reassure her constantly. We all climbed into Jessica's truck looking like zombies.

We arrived 30 minutes early waiting in an empty hospital lobby in nervous silence before Nurse Laura arrived. She led us to the family waiting room outside of the surgical room. She called us *Team Al* as most donors only have one family member. Al had three to support her.

Nurse Laura was covered with official looking ID cards with different colored lanyards and held a small white and orange cooler. I looked over at Jessica and asked, "What is the cooler for?" She explained Nurse Laura was the first in a chain of command, responsible for being in surgery with Al, certifying that the collected bone marrow was put in the cooler. She would then hand carry the cooler to the next chain of command, a courier who would special transport the cooler to the hospital where the baby would have the transplant. Jessica said the doctor told her the baby would have the procedure done in the United States but that is all we were allowed to know.

Al got up to change, smiling while giving us a small cheery wave. Nurse Laura came back in almost an hour and told us we could come into the pre operative room to give a last hug before surgery. *Team Al* was not prepared for what happened next.

Tommy, Jessica and I rounded the corner from the family waiting room to the pre operative area into a heartbreaking scene. A tiny fragile girl in one of those horrible hospital gowns sat in a large plastic chair in a cold room filled with medical equipment. Her entire body was trembling, her face frozen in fear, her eyes brimming with tears. She was absolutely terrified.

Jessica moved toward her and they cried out, struggling against each other in a death grip. Tommy calmly reassured them, reminding me of Russell Crowe in the *Gladiator,* helping soldiers prepare for battle. They broke apart and Tommy comforted Al as she clutched his arm at the shoulder. I kissed her cheek while suppressing my urge to go into rescue mode, wanting to pick her up and run out of the hospital, imagining Nurse Laura chasing me with the little orange and white cooler. Instead of the rescue, Nurse Laura said, "It is time" and motioned Al toward the operating room.

As they walked away in slow motion, I stood next to Jessica and stared. Al stopped, slowly turning around in front of two large metal doors that would swing open into the operating room. I blinked as she looked back at us, through blurry tears I saw a shimmering angel with blue hair reflecting off the metal with a halo like glow, completely around her. She slowly turned back around and walked through those doors. Jessica burst into tears.

Tommy steered Jessica around the corner into the waiting room and sat her down. I found Kleenex for her and sat down next to her. Tommy sat down right next to me, like a guard dog. There was lots of room in the empty waiting room, plenty of other seats but the three of us piled together like glue. Jessica never stopped crying, she did not make any noise but the tears never stopped flowing down her cheeks.

We sat there for a few hours, Tommy getting up once, quickly getting Jessica a Coke, returning swiftly to his guard dog position. I stared at the picture of sunflowers on the wall. I wondered if Al's bone marrow would be able to save this baby. Maybe the parents of the baby would be able to enjoy raising their child who could grow up to have children and maybe those children would have children. I slowly realized Al had the ability to change the world. There is not a way for the family of the baby to pay Al for what she was doing in that operating room, she was giving them a priceless gift.

Jessica started to email family to update them on Al as she continued to cry. The air still had that steely feel and now I felt a rawness to it. I started to write this story. Jessica saw me writing fast and furious and asked if I was taking a class. I smiled and thought the class I am taking today no school could teach. This was life.

Suddenly, Nurse Laura burst out of the operating room running around the corner into the family waiting room gripping the cooler. She shouted, "She did fine!" pushing the heavy glass doors open and running down the hall. Our eyes were wide as we watched her sprint with all those ID tags swirling around her like an octopus. Jessica choked and whispered, "I wonder if they are taking Al's bone marrow to a baby at my children's hospital?" She burst into tears, this time loudly, but these were tears of relief.

We sat back down in shock mode, still sitting too close to each other. Jessica started to fumble with her phone, trying to figure out how to call her husband when the doctor came in, a regal man with grey hair in a white coat. Jessica jumped up; he put his hand on her shoulder and smiled. Jessica exclaimed "Twenty two minutes!" and hugged him. She said, "Al was under general anesthesia for only 22 minutes, they were able to get all the bone marrow they needed!"

I marveled that Al could possibly save a life in 22 minutes. The doctor told Jessica that Al may never know the baby, but he will tell her if the donation worked. Al was out of recovery, moved to a hospital room for observation for the day. I felt utter joy, the raw steely air was gone, and the sun was shining through a window. I watched sea gulls flying by in what looked like a playful dance.

Team Al sat there in the hospital room looking at Al with silly smiles on our faces. For some reason, we were acting ridiculously goofy. Al was in pain but laughing and joking at us, you would never know she just had an operation. They had drilled a hole in both of her hipbones!

Jessica and I leaned back in our chairs and watched Tommy, both of us very relaxed as we admired his nursing skills. Tommy attended to Al's every need, feeding her Jello, making her sip tea, adjusting her blankets and the red hospital socks on her feet. We made it back to the hotel in the afternoon without a hitch, Al and Tommy decided to take a nap. No matter the outcome of the surgery, I know Al would do it all over again. Al knows in her heart she did her best to help a child like the ones walking the halls at the children's hospital.

Jessica and I went to the hotel restaurant for dinner where we talked for hours, not going to bed until the wee hours of the night. One thing I have figured out about angels from this experience. They do not know they are angels. They think they are just people.

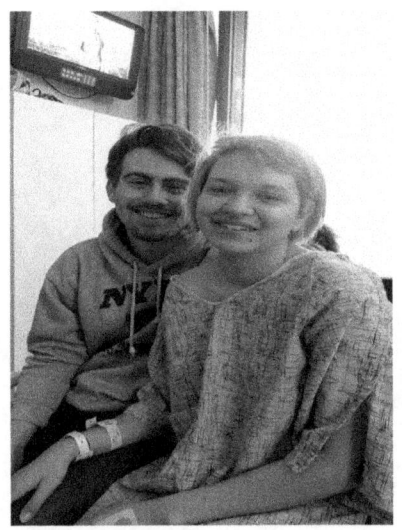

Tommy and Al